Maman, Tell Me My Story One More Time

Mélanie Dumas

Library and Archives Canada Cataloguing in Publication

CIP data on file with the National Library and Archives

ISBN 978-1-926582-94-8

For Oklyn and Koraly

My Dear Oklyn and My Dear Koraly,

What you are about to read is my gift to you. It is your story, the story of two courageous girls who fought for their lives. It is also a story of two girls who, at such a young age, taught so much to their parents about life, love and friendship. Writing the true stories of your births and doing it in my second language was not something I would have thought possible a couple of years ago. But after you came into my life, I felt I had to write this story so that you would understand where we are coming from and would feel the love your Daddy and I have for both of you. You will find that it is a sad story at times, but remember that it is also one of hope for families who are going through the same difficulties we experienced.

Now that our feelings of fear related to your births have been replaced by the joy of witnessing you grow, I can tell you that there is nothing more rewarding for me as looking at both of you developing and becoming your own little people. When I hear your daily new words, Oklyn, or see your toothless smile, Koraly, or when both of you just get so excited to see me after a long night's sleep, to me this is just pure pleasure, pure joy. In essence, happiness. Can life get any better than that?

As I am writing this, you are still very young and you have a long life ahead of you. Make sure that you make it as beautiful as you are, and that you never forget that the battle for your lives that you fought for many months while in the hospital makes you deserve a special place in this big, big world.

Love,
Maman

Surprise, I am Here!

June 22nd, 2008 is a date that I will never forget. How could I? It will be a joyful day every year when we will celebrate my oldest daughter's birthday, but it will also be a day when I will take the time to reflect, and remember how everything in my life changed. Anyone who goes from being happily married and living the high life with no children to having a baby would probably make the same statement. Children do change your life! But in some cases, the journey on which you are about to embark when you first see your little bundle of joy can be a very traumatic experience that will leave a scar for the rest of your life. The story I am about to tell is not all that pretty, but it is the truth. I wanted to share this experience so that my daughters will know their story and will understand how fortunate we are that things turned out so well for all of us. I also wanted to tell this story so that new parents encountering difficulties with the birth of their children would see that there is hope ahead, and beautiful days as well. But along with hope, parents need to face the reality that this birth may also bring tears, fears and disappointments. So here is the story of my beautiful daughters, told in an honest and humble way.

A few years ago, I would have admitted to being afraid of hospitals and being afraid of getting sick. To me, hospitals were not a happy place. Do people ever get good news when they need to visit a hospital? I believed hospitals were for older people, unfortunate people and, truthfully, people who were just neglecting their health and making poor decisions. On June 22nd, 2008, it took only a few hours for me to change this belief that I had had about the hospital, because the hospital would become part of my life and even a place I would call home.

Beginning this story on the day of the delivery would be unrealistic as it would not recall all the excitement that led to the actual event. In reality, it started when my husband Mackenzie and I met. I was born and raised in a French-speaking town of about a thousand people. After finishing my teaching degree and looking for a little adventure, I moved to an Anglophone city called Everwood, a city of about 80,000 people. Although I often return to my hometown for visits, I find it hard to believe that I left more than a decade ago. I ended up falling in love with the English language, finding a great job as a French Immersion teacher and also falling in love with a wonderful man. As for Mack, this wonderful man, he was also born in a different city and even in a different province than the one where we are presently living. He fell in love with the lifestyle that he found here and the freedom that his job brought to his life as a replay technician for sports. His work gives him the opportunity to work anywhere in the province or country where there is a televised event. He mainly works in Voulder, a bigger centre of about 2,000,000 people. This story begins about a year before we got pregnant, when we decided that an addition to the family would be something that would bring us love, joy and fun times. Let's just say that year gave us time for practice and for mastering the art of procreating! Finally, on January 4th, 2008, feeling a little lucky, I bought a pregnancy test, definitely not the first one, and to my absolute surprise, joy and terror I discovered something amazing. It finally had worked. We were pregnant! I spent the afternoon of January 4th visualizing the next nine months. First, we decided that we would not tell anybody until the 12th week of the pregnancy. That decision didn't even last twenty-four hours. We were just so excited! By the time I went back to work after the Christmas break on January 7th, everybody I cared about knew of the exciting news. I was already sharing my nightmares of delivering a ten-pound baby, Mack's size when he was born.

I had the perfect picture of my baby, one with chubby little rosy cheeks and an angelic smile. I had imagined every detail of the pregnancy! I had in mind that I would be sick for the first three months, would be glowing and full of energy for the next three to four months and would get huge and exhausted from carrying the extra weight over the last month. That was to be the sequence of events of this perfect pregnancy. I was positive that with all that careful planning, we had it all figured out! Being pregnant was going to be the easy part of this whole new adventure. Sure, I had my little superstitions. For example, just to be on the safe side I wasn't going to buy any baby things, paint the baby's room, or change anything in the house for the new little one until at least the sixth month of the pregnancy. Yes, I was sick a couple of times in the first twelve weeks. Yes, I did feel like I was glowing and was full of energy at some point, but I never had time to get that big round belly because at twenty-seven weeks and four days our bundle of joy had a whole other agenda! Eager to see the world, she made her grand entrance. But it wasn't the entrance we had hoped for!

It was the previous Monday afternoon that I started noticing that something was going on. When putting my sandals back on after spending the day under the sun at a friend's house, I realized that my feet were very swollen and my sandals were not fitting me anymore. I shook my head and blamed it on sitting all afternoon in the sun. Or maybe it was that ham I had eaten for lunch that was probably too salty for a pregnant woman. I thought that putting my feet up for a couple of hours would remedy the problem. This did indeed seem to solve the problem. Or was it just that my eyes were getting used to the look of my swollen feet and that had I forgotten what my feet looked like normally? How was I supposed to know any better? On Wednesday night it was clear that something was wrong when I started to have severe intermittent back and abdominal pain. Beginning to feel concerned, I went online to find out if all of this was normal. I clicked on "pregnancy and back pain" and found that this could be an early sign of labour. I thought, "Here I am starting labour and I am sitting at home by myself!" I hadn't had any contractions, but I was still concerned that something was going on, so I drove myself to the hospital because Mack was away working, and saw the on-call maternity doctor. After a quick exam, he told me that I was not in labour and that nothing was about to happen. I was relieved, to say the least, and happy to be reassured that heartburn and back pain are very common in pregnancy. Tums tablets could help relieve those symptoms. The doctor also told me that there was a possibility that I had strained my back and that lying down and watching television would put me back on my feet in no time. Feeling happy with this information, I stopped at a gas station on the way home to buy Ibuprofen to cure my bad headache, and made my way home to get a much-needed rest. To my surprise, the Ibuprofen did not cure the headache and the heartburn wasn't going away with the prescribed Tums tablets. But I finally fell asleep and when I woke up the next day I was feeling better.

I started to be concerned again that something was going on when my friend told me that my face reminded her of the Pacman character – round and fat. It was, apparently, quite swollen. Again I tried to find an excuse for all of this so I blamed it on that ham sandwich I had eaten the previous Monday and on the fact that I hadn't been drinking enough water. I was, by then, being careful with my sodium intake as I thought for sure that the swelling had all been caused by the salty ham. But after giving it some serious thought, I started to question what was really going on with me. Every day something new and wrong was asking for my attention – swollen feet, back pain, abdominal pain, headache, vomiting, even a difference in the odour of my urine. However, all of these could just be the symptoms of a normal pregnancy. I was not terribly worried, but I still didn't feel well enough to do much around the house, exercise or go out with friends. People around me were starting to tell me that something was amiss and that if I was not able to do these activities, I was probably ill. Well, I was extremely ill and what I didn't know was that I was putting myself and my baby in danger with every passing minute, and that delivery of my baby would be the only cure for all these problems that I was experiencing. I made another trip to the Emergency ward of the hospital early Saturday evening. This time Mack was with me. Usually, when a pregnant woman is past twenty weeks they send her up to Obstetrics, but with me they chose to tend to me right there in the Emergency ward. This time I was told that all I had was severe heartburn. They also told me that pregnancy does often bring uncomfortable symptoms and I should just "suck it up."

More than an hour after taking the medication given to me at the hospital, I was still feeling very ill. I was having trouble breathing, trouble walking, trouble standing up straight. I was feeling acute pain all over my body. I was "sucking it up" as much as I could, but there was a limit to what a pregnant woman can endure so I made my way to the hospital for a third time that week. I was finally sent to the third floor, the Obstetrics floor. While I was telling a nurse about my symptoms, a visiting obstetrician from the Voulder General Hospital passed by and overheard me. She knew why my body was slowly shutting down. She told me what I didn't want to hear: in order to save my life and the life of my baby girl, we would have to deliver this baby immediately. Not only was I suffering from a pregnancy disease called preeclampsia, but I was also a victim of "Hemolysis, Elevated Liver Enzymes and Low Platelets Syndrome" (HELLP), which occurs in roughly 5% of women who get preeclampsia. She told me that the Everwood Queen's Hospital was not equipped to care for a baby born at only twenty-seven weeks. We needed to go to a hospital that had been designated as a "level three". Talk about luck! I had so many questions at that moment. Was this baby completely formed? Was this baby going to be healthy? Would she survive? How heavy was she at this moment? Was the Everwood Queen's Hospital (EQH) equipped well enough to handle a fragile baby? Was the staff qualified enough? Did they have adequate specialists? Was I going to be all right? Were we going to be well cared for at the next hospital? "Where were we going?" was the next question. One minute we were going to Voulder, a minute later we were going to Ablington, then Crescent and even Laurier was a strong possibility. These hospitals were situated in cities with populations of over a million people. What was going on? Our baby girl needed a bed and I needed one as well, because both of us were in danger. Finding two available empty beds was not an easy task.

It would be wrong to say that I clearly understood what was going on at that time. I felt numb. It was just too much! Yes, I felt very sick, but I didn't necessarily think that delivering my baby was the right thing to do at that moment. It was all happening so fast. Over the next fifteen minutes, I was told to strip and lie down, my blood pressure was taken every five minutes, a catheter was inserted in my bladder, and an intravenous of magnesium sulphate was started in my arm. I was asked to swallow a number of pills, I underwent numerous blood tests and I was given a steroid injection. Most of this was done to avoid the seizure that could be caused by my escalating high blood pressure. It was also being done to help my baby girl have the best possible start that she could at the tender age of twenty-seven weeks and four days.

At this point, I started to have an inkling of what was really happening. I was hearing words like seizure, kidney failure and liver failure. I was also hearing names of medications which were sounding quite familiar. Suddenly it hit me! My mom who had suffered from a stroke ten years ago had been prescribed these medications, Adalat and Labetalol, and is taking them to this day. Was I about to have a stroke? I was not able to ask any coherent questions and even if I had, I might not have understood the answers. Doctors were sent in, one after another, to keep me informed of what was about to happen. First the obstetrician who was going to perform the caesarean-section came in with the blood results and confirmed that this disease was causing a great deal of distress to both the baby and myself. She informed us that we would be air-evacuated as soon as an Infant Transport team coming from the city of Voulder became available and two beds at Voulder General Hospital could be found. She was sorry to tell us that if the team were not able to make it on time to save our lives, the caesarean-section would have to be performed in Everwood. Everwood Queen's Hospital would have to deliver a baby of twenty-seven weeks and four days. That in itself was worrisome to me. It wasn't that I didn't trust EQH and their specialists, but I could not imagine a small hospital like Everwood having the necessary equipment to handle this life-and-death situation. Then the news came that the Infant Transport team was not able to make it on time. The delivery was indeed going to take place in Everwood. The Infant Transport team would instead come some time the next day to pick us up and take us to the Voulder General hospital. I was in pain but the pain was endurable, so I felt there was no need to panic just yet. Minutes later, all the doctors followed each other into the hospital room to inform us about premature babies, c-sections, undergoing anesthesia, and the HELLP syndrome. I felt as though I was in a bad movie. All of the doctors had foreign accents. A couple of months later I was told they were from Russia, South Africa, and various parts of Asia. This, together with the fact that I was a French Canadian myself living in an Anglophone community, was making the situation even more difficult for me to understand.

Four hours after I was admitted to the Everwood hospital, a couple of nurses wheeled me to the operating room where I was welcomed by the obstetrician, my family doctor, the anesthetist and two nurses from the Neonatal Intensive Care Unit who would be assisting the paediatrician once the baby was born. To say the least, I was very confused by the number of specialists coming for the delivery. I kept thinking that I was about to give birth to a twenty-seven week and four-day old baby without my husband to hold my hand. Also that the most wonderful day of my life, the day that I had been anticipating for so long, was going to become a nightmare. I was about to embark on a journey that I didn't choose, and I was feeling assaulted with all the information that was being passed on to me.

What happened from four a.m., the time that Oklyn was born, until eleven a.m. is still a mystery to me. I wish I could describe the birth of our baby girl, but I can't recall anything because of the anesthetic. I read reports and Mack gave me updates but I am still not positive about exactly what happened within the walls of the NICU once Oklyn was transferred there from the operating room. Did I want to know? No, I didn't! I remember hearing scary words like resuscitation, cerebral hemorrhage and chronic lung disease. I was slowly getting answers to my earlier questions. Was she going to be all right? The answers were hitting me so fast and furious that I began to experience something quite unexpected. I was feeling afraid of my own baby daughter. I was afraid to see her, afraid even to be told about her. I just wanted to turn back the clock, go back home and let her grow where she belonged, in my comfy belly. After the morphine had set in we were air-evacuated to the General Hospital in Voulder. It was a sunny Sunday morning plane ride that I will always remember, the plane ride that separated Oklyn and me until I was able to find the strength to go and visit her in the NICU. The sky was a beautiful blue, there was no sight of a storm approaching, but inside I was hearing rumbling thunder and seeing streaks of lightning.

The trip didn't take long, and after a short ambulance ride I was admitted to the Voulder General Hospital. Oklyn was also admitted, but to the Voulder General Children's

Hospital. Our two hospitals were located in the same building. Voulder General Hospital was very foreign to me. I hadn't known that Voulder General Hospital was a teaching hospital, so I was taken aback to see not one, but six doctors come into my room. I finally had to concede that the Everwood Queen's Hospital had been telling the truth and that I was very ill. The Voulder General Hospital is an academic health centre affiliated with a couple of universities in the Voulder area, so doctors were always accompanied by intern students. Here I was lying in a bed, recounting my past week to six attentive doctors. I don't remember what I told them. The morphine was working well on me and I didn't even know where I was, who I was and why I was giving a speech to six doctors. I was drugged up and just a mess, but trying as hard as I could to keep it together. I was still shocked at what was happening and why I had to deliver my baby so early. Again I just wanted to be home to peacefully enjoy the last three months of my pregnancy. To confirm the Everwood doctors' diagnosis, the Voulder doctors ordered the tests to be redone. The test results confirmed that the Everwood doctors had been correct. The obstetrician-on-call had saved my life and the life of my little Oklyn. But where was Oklyn? I thought about asking, but since I didn't know anything about this hospital and because I was not confident that I could handle the truth, I kept the question to myself.

The hours that followed were busy. Although I was told I needed rest, there was always someone coming to my room to take my blood, give me a blood test result, give me pills to swallow, take my blood pressure, do a physical exam or introduce me to breast pumping because my little Oklyn was apparently going to need colostrum to get through her difficult start. “So,” I thought, “Oklyn must be alive if they want me to provide her with milk.” But I was not going to ask for fear of hearing that yes, she was alive but severely handicapped. Mack was still on his way driving from Everwood to Voulder, so he couldn’t answer my questions. Once more I just tried to keep it together and do what I had been told to do, which was to pump my breasts eight times a day to get the milk flowing.

The hospital staff explained that I was a patient in a hospital in Voulder and was seriously ill. I was stressed and still not totally understanding what had happened, but at least one thing had changed for the better. Here at the Voulder General Hospital I was not seeing the worried look that I had seen in the eyes of the Everwood doctors. Here, the doctors were making me believe that they knew what they were doing and that it was the best place for me to be. I still wasn’t feeling calm, because I was still not sure if I would survive all of this, but the competent staff reassured me with the information that the HELLP syndrome is a curable disease if treated early enough by specialists.

Mack arrived at the hospital about an hour after Oklyn and I did. It was a relief to have him there to share the weight of this ordeal. In between pumping and trying to comprehend this nightmare, I was hearing a few things about Oklyn when doctors and nurses would ask Mack how she was doing. I was not getting much information except that she was 840 grams at birth, one pound and thirteen ounces. The strange phenomenon of feeling afraid of my own baby girl was intensifying. As the hours wore on, I was becoming more and more afraid of Oklyn. In my mind there was no way that she would survive, so there was no point even talking about her. The phone started to ring, the e-mails started to fill up our mailboxes, the presents started to arrive, but I was just numb to all of this. I didn't want to have anything to do with any of it. Why were people sending me congratulation cards or e-mails? After all, I had almost died and killed my baby girl! Was this supposed to be a happy moment? I thought I didn't deserve all of this attention! I still wanted to be at home sitting on the couch eating a bagel, one of my biggest cravings throughout the twenty-seven weeks of my pregnancy. Why was this happening to me?

Our friends and family were understandably anxious to hear all our news, so Mack sent an e-mail to announce the birth of Oklyn and inform everyone of the unusual circumstances. Here it is.

Hello Everyone,

As some of you know, Melanie gave birth by caesarean on Sunday morning at 4:03 am in Everwood. We went into the hospital late on Saturday night with what we thought was bad heartburn. After getting some medication and going home, the "heartburn" got much worse and we went back to the hospital and it became apparent that it was not heartburn. There were a few things that troubled the doctors, including preeclampsia and what we now know to be the HELLP syndrome. It was decided that they needed to get the baby out as Melanie's health was now seriously at risk. They were able to give Melanie a steroid shot in order to start boosting the baby's lung abilities and after some time for this to take effect, Melanie was prepped for surgery (4:00am). She went under general anesthesia and the doctors delivered a baby girl at twenty-seven weeks and four days. After Oklyn was breathing I went with her to the NICU where we stayed for several hours while they monitored her and stabilized her for transport. Melanie was able to come in at about 7:30am to see the little one and then I went with her back to her room to recover and get stabilized as well. At 11:00 am both Melanie and Oklyn were sent via airplane to Voulder General Hospital. I drove down and we were back together at about 14:30 pm. Everything to this point has gone extremely well, considering the circumstances. Melanie was taken off all her IVs and is now able to move around a bit. She has started with the breast pump and we are making milk deliveries to the NICU for them to give to Oklyn. Oklyn has been stable now since about 5:30 am Sunday morning and at this point they say that is very good. She is breathing room air with ease and there is talk of taking her off the ventilator as early as tomorrow. Also they will be doing an ultrasound on her head to see if there is any brain damage that may have occurred.

She is small, very small, just under two pounds and about fifteen inches long, but VERY cute with a little hair and a big toe that Melanie says she wants to bite. We will be staying at the Voulder General Hospital for the next few days at Arbutus Ward room 6. After Melanie is well, we will probably head back to the condo where we will station ourselves until Oklyn gets transferred back to Everwood. No word yet as to when that may happen. Thank you for all the thoughts and well wishes that you have sent. Melanie is looking forward to seeing and talking to everyone but as she is still needing lots of rest to recover from the surgery, she may not get to everyone right away.

I'll try to keep everyone updated as things move along.

Mélanie, Mack and Oklyn

Mack's e-mail was great, but of course it didn't stop people from wanting to get in touch with us. I ignored many phone calls by asking Mack to tell my friends that I was busy talking to a nurse or a doctor, or that I was sleeping, or just not by the phone. I spoke only to my parents, my sister, and my friend Lynn as I felt obligated to give them an update. I was not sure what to tell them because I didn't know much about what was happening myself, so I tried to avoid the topic and instead I'd ask them how things were going with them. One was renovating her house, one was training for a half-marathon, my parents were enjoying the warm season so I just kept asking questions about their lives, trying to avoid what was going on in mine.

I was obviously not the first mom going along that route and after about forty-eight hours post delivery, a few nurses were starting to see that I was in denial. They knew that I needed to face reality and go visit Oklyn in the NICU. I kept saying that I would go but I didn't, because I was afraid of what that reality was going to be. I was blaming it on the fact that I was sick and weak, but in truth my health was slowly improving and my body was giving signs that it would pass through this ordeal without too much damage. I was told that I was going to be transferred from the emergency room to a recovery room upstairs. I was strongly encouraged to personally deliver the colostrum that I was getting from pumping my breasts to Oklyn. It was time! I was about to put on my Supermom's cape for the first time and go visit her.

An Unknown World

Sitting in a wheelchair being pushed by Mack, I was making my way into what I would describe as a foreign world, the world of Neonatal. The walls were painted bright yellow. Stars and moons were drawn on a colorful blue floor. Lions, giraffes, elephants and cows covered a strip of wallpaper glued to the wall. A first glance made me believe that things were going to be okay, but the second one brought me back to reality and to why I was there. As I approached Oklyn's bedside I felt like my five senses were being violated all at once. There was the smell of the hospital, the sight of computers, ventilators, fake fantasy, the sound of the alarm letting the staff know they needed to have a closer look at one of their patients, a bad aftertaste that I still have when I fear something could happen to my girls, and the touch of nothing. There was no-one to hold and cuddle with. I was starting to get the feeling that what was happening inside the walls of the NICU was far from a fairy tale.

Oklyn's nurse, a beautiful young Asian girl, greeted me

with a warm smile. She reassured me that things were fine, even though Oklyn's incubator was covered completely with a quilt. My baby, apparently, was sensitive to the light. There was only so much a new mom could handle. I started to cry, cry and cry. Looking at me compassionately, the nurse paged the doctor so he could come and discuss all of my concerns. But what concerns? I hadn't come with concerns. I had just been stopping by to deliver the colostrum I had been pumping for my baby. The doctor arrived quickly and told us that Oklyn was doing just fine. Was he kidding me? I thought, "If he's describing Oklyn we're not speaking about the same baby." To me, a fine baby meant a term baby. A baby breathing on her own, a baby that you could put to the breast right after delivery, a baby that you could hold as often as you wanted and as long as you wanted, a baby that would bring you joy at first sight. I understood later that the doctor meant that she was doing fine for her gestational age, but there was still going to be a long road ahead before I could describe her as fine.

Then the nurse took the quilt off the incubator to properly introduce me to Oklyn. But where was Oklyn? A closer peek was going to make me fall apart. Oklyn was about as big as my hand and was connected with tubes from head to toe. Her pretty face was covered by a giant mask called a "continuous positive airway pressure" (CPAP) machine. That was it; I could not take it any longer. The bright and joyful colors of that room were suddenly fading, and inside my mind it was growing darker and darker. As I was getting wheeled out of the NICU to go get some rest, I passed by some parents who were giving me sympathetic looks and weak smiles. On the left side of Oklyn's incubator was a dad holding his son and singing to him. A month later I found out that his little baby boy had been hospitalised for six months already and that his adventure at the hospital would last more than a year. To the right of Oklyn there was a crying mom whose baby boy with Down's Syndrome was needing heart surgery. She was talking to the surgeon and needed the help of a translator because she could only speak Mandarin. I wondered if the translator was really there because of a language problem or to provide emotional support, because the mom was in denial just as I was.

When I got upstairs to my new room, I was again welcomed by a very friendly nurse. By now, the Voulder General Hospital felt safe and kind to me because there they had all the answers I needed. My bedroom was big, but almost too big because despite how safe I felt there, I also felt lonely. Because my health was improving, I was not getting all the attention that I had been given when I was first admitted. The nurses were still checking me every four hours for blood pressure, blood tests, pain and medication. There was the odd conversation about Oklyn, but because I was very quiet and very brief in my responses to their questions, the exchanges were short. My emotions were alternating from feeling very sad to very angry. I was positive that I had done everything necessary to give birth to a healthy baby. It was making me angry to see other new moms going outside for a cigarette or to hear that there was a wing for moms who had abused illicit substances during their pregnancy. I, on the other hand, had done everything right. I was so upset and I couldn't understand why working out at the gym, eating healthily, and getting enough rest didn't allow me to have a cuddly, healthy, bouncing baby girl.

Mack was never too far away from me and was keeping me updated about Oklyn. Whenever I was by myself I was lost in my thoughts. I didn't really see the point of visiting Oklyn because I didn't believe she would survive. We were welcome to visit Oklyn as much as we wanted and at any time we wanted. The doors of the NICU were always open for the parents, but I didn't go because I was afraid to get attached to someone I believed I would lose. I was still pumping eight times a day to provide milk for Oklyn. I was told to act like she was with me, so I was waking up at night for regular "night feedings" just as if she was there in the room with me. During the nights I would be awakened by babies crying in the other rooms. I would see dads walking their babies around the hallway to help them fall asleep after their feedings. Mack had no one to hold and no reason to walk the hallway. Instead he opted to wash the pump parts and take the milk to the fridge at the front desk. He was keeping it together and staying strong for me, but I wondered if inside he was falling apart as much as I was.

While in the hospital, we started to get into a regular routine, or I should say Mack did. He would get up in the morning, go visit Oklyn and attend the rounds. The rounds are an opportunity for parents to listen to what the doctors are saying about their child. Parents can ask questions and express their concerns. After rounds, Mack would come back and relay what he had heard. He would try to cheer me up by telling me stories about other babies who seemed to be in worse shape than ours. He would tell me about babies with heart disease, infections, cerebral hemorrhages and necrotizing enterocolitis, a serious complication of prematurity. The neonatal world was a world filled with nothing but sadness.

Friends and family continued to e-mail and give us their support wherever the help was needed. We had left Everwood so quickly that many things had been left unattended. They were also calling to set up visitations. The NICU's doors were open for friends and family only if the parents approved their visit. My reaction to their kind thoughts might be difficult to understand. As much as I needed their support, it was making me furious that they wanted to come and visit Oklyn and me. I thought they wanted to see Oklyn just so that they would see how tiny she was. She was not a freak show; she was a sick baby who, in my mind, was not even going to survive. Mack, on the other hand, was eager to have them visit. I think he just wanted us to be normal. After all, it is the normal thing for friends and family to go to the hospital to visit newborns. Here we were having people visiting us, just like normal. But I was still very afraid to see Oklyn so I did not accompany them, nor would I ask them questions or discuss what they had seen.

Our first good news arrived on Thursday, June 26th. There was an ultrasound done on Oklyn's head to check for an intraventricular hemorrhage, and the result came back normal. Oklyn didn't have bleeding in the brain, and her brain looked normal. I will always remember the look Mack and I exchanged when the doctor came all the way upstairs to tell us the good news. That was, and still is, the best high five I've ever given and have ever received. For the first time in almost a week I thought there was an angel somewhere who had been taking care of Oklyn and me on that June 22nd. Hope turned into a little slice of reality.

I was still not visiting Oklyn much and when I was visiting her, I still didn't dare to look at her too closely. I was, however, getting more familiar with the NICU. Other moms began to approach us and share their similar experiences. Doctors were answering my questions and researchers were ready with information. There were many studies being done at the Voulder General Hospital. The Magnetic Resonance Imaging (MRI) study was one that interested us, so we enrolled Oklyn. An MRI was going to be performed on her to measure her brain structure and detect any possible injury. On one hand, I was petrified to get the results of this MRI, but on the other hand, I thought that this test could give us insight into questions we had been asking since her birth. The results came back normal! Oklyn's brain was developing normally. There was a chance that things were going to be all right.

The day came when I was healthy enough to be discharged. Oklyn, however, would need to stay in the hospital a while longer. My health was not 100%, but I was well enough to be sent home. I still needed to have my blood pressure monitored every second day. We were lucky to have family who owned a condominium in downtown Voulder. The commute between the hospital and home was a short jaunt. Mack was very happy for us to leave the hospital as he was looking forward to living in the condo and regaining some privacy. I, on the other hand, was afraid to leave the hospital as it meant I was not going to live under the same roof as my baby girl. Our last visit to see Oklyn before being discharged was a cruel one. I have seen how exhilarated new parents usually leave the hospital proudly carrying their beautiful new bundles of joy, but our exit was just the opposite. In my perfect plan, I would have been walking out slowly because of the pain from delivery. Mack would have been at my side, carrying all the presents that we'd received in one hand and in the other, a car seat where our new little addition would be safely resting. But the only thing I remember carrying that day were prescriptions that had to be filled out because I now needed to take eleven pills just to get through the day. After telling Oklyn that we would be back for a visit that night, we made our way to the car to drive to the condo. It was a very quiet ride home, with me sobbing the whole way. This was not working well for me. I didn't want to be away from Oklyn now; I wanted her to be with us. It is hard to explain how in just one week my feelings had changed from being so scared of Oklyn to not wanting to leave her at the hospital. At the time, I thought I felt that way because I was becoming a mom who just wanted the best for her baby girl. I also thought only her mom could give her the best nurturing she needed at the time.

Here is an e-mail that I sent to let friends and family know that I was now discharged.

Well, it has been an eventful week for Mack, Oklyn and myself. I have many questions without answers and it's hard to think that at this time last

Saturday I was working out at the gym. Mack and I are now home (as much as home can be for me in Voulder) and as you already know, Oklyn will be staying at the Voulder General Children's Hospital for the next little while.

We would like to thank all of you for your support, beautiful flowers, food baskets, phone calls, e-mails... We needed your support and we are very thankful for having so many great friends from everywhere. Thank you! The road seems very long until Oklyn can come home, but we will stay strong.

The staff at the Voulder General Children's Hospital is amazing. They are here for us and we can count on them to give us great support. Oklyn is doing fine and is apparently developing by the book for a premature baby. That means that what is happening with her right now is not surprising any doctors here. This is very good news.

We will keep you posted over the next few weeks and please feel free to call us and stop by if you are in the Voulder area over the summer.

For people who didn't get Mack's e-mails because you were only on my list of friends and are still wondering what happened to me, I was diagnosed with preeclampsia, but I was also a victim of the HELLP syndrome, which occurs in roughly 5% of women who get preeclampsia. Talk about luck!!! I would also like to say it was not because of my short cervix. It was totally bad luck and it doesn't mean that I would have this happening over a sec-

ond pregnancy. Not that we are even thinking about this right now.

One more thing and it is for the mommies group: I remember all of you telling me about your stories when you gave birth. I remember sitting there and thinking that giving birth is quite a scary thing and can be very traumatic. I can't wait to attend the next dinner and talk to you about my experience. It will be about having many doctors around me in the operating room, being transported by air ambulance, having to talk with doctors from Russia, South Africa, Asia and not understanding anything because of their accent. I will wait for that dinner to bring up the near stroke I almost had as it would be too scary to tell on an e-mail.

Thanks again for all of your generous support.

Mélanie

Mack went back to work the Monday after I was discharged. After all, I didn't need help at home to take care of Oklyn. My days were spent at the hospital pumping and staring at Oklyn's incubator. I would sit beside the incubator and just wait for something to happen. I would also use that time to read about premature babies and to try to learn more about all the new medical terms that I was hearing in the NICU. It was good for me to read. It was keeping my mind active, but it was also causing abnormal sleeplessness at night as I would start worrying about everything that could go wrong.

Oklyn's progress in the NICU was as the doctor first described it to us. He told us that Oklyn would take two steps forward and one step back. She was very much following that pattern. There were days when she was doing very well and when I was finally able to smile and enjoy being a new mom, but there were other days when I was brought back to the sad reality of the NICU. Every setback that Oklyn experienced felt like someone was stabbing me deeper and deeper each time. There were many days that just waking up in the morning was a difficult task to do. I was constantly sad and depressed. Mack was very good at making me feel like a new mom. He took care of buying everything a new mom would need - breastfeeding bras, breast pads and even nipple cream. He was the one spending the most time with me and he noticed that I was just not myself since Oklyn's birth. He suggested that I consult a psychiatrist to deal with all my confused feelings relating to this event. I was willing to do this because I knew that I was not acting as my usual self. It was good for me to talk to the psychiatrist about how I was feeling. She specialized in postpartum depression, and I felt like she knew and understood what I was going through. But she didn't diagnose me with postpartum depression. Instead, she thought that I was going through normal feelings of guilt, loss and disappointment. My feelings matched her description, but it was upsetting to realise that she would not be able to cure me. There was no quick fix. It was overwhelming to me that in order to feel better I would have to do the work, and that work was to talk about the ordeal to friends and family. I didn't know where to start, though, so I just brushed all these feelings aside and kept doing what seemed to be the most important thing at the time, which was to visit Oklyn and wait for something to happen.

Although it helped to see the psychiatrist, it wasn't an instant cure. Mack tried other things to make me feel better as a new mom. During the daily hospital rounds, he asked if I would be able to go later and hold Oklyn the way many other parents were doing. It's hard to believe that in these entire ten days since my baby girl had been born, I hadn't yet actually held her. In the NICU, there is a procedure called "skin to skin." The premature baby is held in an upright position on the mom's bare chest - tummy to tummy, in between the breasts. The doctors and nurses agreed that Oklyn was stable enough for me to do this. Even after being told that the medical, physical, and emotional benefits for both of us were going to be advantageous, I was very nervous to do a "skin to skin" with Oklyn. I felt that she was too fragile for this and I knew that if something were to go wrong from my holding her I would never forgive myself. After being assured that it was a common practice in the NICU, I agreed to give it a try.

Holding Oklyn for the first time was an amazing experience. Her ten-day-old little body felt warm, soft and surprisingly not that fragile. Suddenly, I experienced a feeling of satisfaction I had not previously thought possible. Oklyn was finally where she belonged, cradled in my arms. This "skin to skin" cuddle was, for me, the first time that I felt like a real mom. At this moment I felt happier than I could have imagined. I really was Oklyn's mom and would be there for her for the rest of my life.

Finally holding Oklyn brought me joy, but at the same time it brought more worries and tears. I felt like Oklyn was going to live and come home with us one day, and this knowledge was making her setbacks harder to take. I was now attached to her, and the fear of losing her from what could happen because of her prematurity was unbearable. She was still fighting for her life, she was still very little, and whenever we would get a phone call from the hospital telling us that Oklyn was having a bad day I would just fall apart and fear the worst. Up until this point, I had been afraid of being with Oklyn. Now I was scared of losing her.

It was on a Friday afternoon, July 18th, that Oklyn surprised me for the first time in her life. Her growing strength had been astonishing me every day, but that particular day when I walked in the nursery I fell in love with her even more. When I got to Oklyn's bedside, the nurse took off the quilt covering her incubator and then, for the first time, I saw her beautiful face without any mask. Oklyn was now breathing on her own! I could finally see that she resembled her dad. She was beautiful! It was weird to look at this little body, not even as big as my two hands, slowly taking big breaths. I started to cry, but this time my tears were finally tears of joy. What a good feeling it was just to sit there and watch her. I spent that afternoon staring at her, but this time I was not lost in my thoughts like I usually was; I was just a proud mom admiring my beautiful baby girl.

At rounds time on Oklyn's thirty-third day of life, they talked about Oklyn transferring to EQH in Everwood where we lived. The doctors thought Oklyn was still frail due to her low weight and her gestational age at birth, but was doing fairly well. They thought she was stable enough to move to a "level two" hospital. I was not prepared for this. I didn't completely trust the Everwood Queen's Hospital. The Emergency doctors there had made a mistake by sending me back home not once but twice with what were very clear signs of preeclampsia. How were they going to properly take care of a baby who weighed barely two pounds? I was also getting accustomed to the Voulder General Children's Hospital. It felt safe to be surrounded by their competent nurses and doctors. It felt reassuring to have the best specialists in the province under the same roof as Oklyn. Mack and I tried to share our concerns with the hospital but the doctors were confident enough to send Oklyn along. I was unsure about the Everwood Queen's Hospital, but because it was also where all my support was, I tried to convince myself that we would be just fine. The Infant Transport Team came to pick up Oklyn and me on her thirty-fifth day of life, July 26th. I left the hospital feeling anxious for what was ahead of us, but while I was walking down the hallway following Oklyn's incubator to get to the ambulance, I swore to myself that, as nice as Voulder General Children's Hospital was, I would never come back. I just wanted to forget this nightmare and have a new start. I was now a new mom with a baby girl who was going to survive and was going to come home and live with us one day.

The neonatal intensive care unit in Everwood Queen's Hospital was not what I had imagined it would be like. It was small and quiet. When we arrived, there were only four nurses in attendance and not a single doctor in sight. I certainly was not used to this, but it didn't feel scary because the nurse who was taking care of the transfer was older and oozed confidence. During her career, she had dealt with many babies sicker than Oklyn. I could sense that she was a caring mom herself and I felt relaxed watching her handle Oklyn. After a few minutes, she introduced me to the pediatrician who would be Oklyn's doctor for the duration of her stay at the hospital. This was not our first introduction, as she had been present the night of the delivery. She could not believe that Oklyn was already back in Everwood and healthy. We exchanged a couple of looks that spoke volumes. I knew what she meant when she described Oklyn as healthy. What she really meant was that Oklyn had escaped having a cerebral hemorrhage. I felt like this doctor and I were somewhat connected to each other because she had been there the day this all started and she was probably the one who had resuscitated Oklyn. After a quick tour of the nursery, I finally took a taxi to my home where I had wanted to be since the beginning of this adventure. This time leaving Oklyn at the hospital didn't seem as difficult as it had the first time we left her at the Voulder General Children's Hospital without me as a patient right next door. This time it felt like she was closer to coming home.

My routine in Everwood was similar to the one in Voulder. I would visit Oklyn three times a day and make sure there was going to be a "skin to skin" cuddle each afternoon. Oklyn was not adjusting well at first and was having numerous daily desaturations. A desaturation is a decrease in the percentage of oxygen found in the circulating blood supply. I was really nervous about these as they would cause the monitor to set off an alarm. A nurse would then come and check Oklyn's breathing, change of colour, and heart rate. There were many false alarms, but other times the nurse would need to stimulate Oklyn to remind her to breathe and even give her oxygen. I was still having a lot of worries and very dark days, but the Everwood Queen's Hospital staff was always able to comfort me.

About three weeks after our transfer to Everwood Queen's Hospital, Oklyn became healthier and steadily gained weight. Her weight gain was slow and there were nights when she was only adding five grams to the scale, but in general she seemed healthier. She was starting to take my milk through bottles and sometimes even on the breast. What a good feeling that was for me to be able to finally feed her. She was not the easiest baby to breastfeed, but her sucking was strong enough. I was now able to do most of the activities related to her care: change her diaper, take her temperature, give her the medication, bathe her, weigh her and feed her. All these tasks seem very easy to do for a new mom, but it's not that easy when you are handling only a three pound baby. Oklyn was now doing well and I was also doing better too! I was back at the gym between my morning and afternoon visits to Oklyn and I was now able to visit friends without having a meltdown. I was starting to enjoy spending time in the nursery as the staff were great and I was not afraid of Oklyn any more. I was able to have a normal conversation and not just talk about Oklyn. I remember liking all the staff and being able to relate to most of them, and was finally able to have friendly chats with them, unlike in Voulder where I could focus only on Oklyn. There was the wine lover, the quilt lover, the dog lover, the

Facebook lover, the Cutie and the Blondie. They were each trying to make Oklyn's stay in the nursery easier on me.

Things were working out for me but I was still very fragile and it was sometimes hard for me to watch new parents take their babies home after a week or two in the nursery. It angered me to see new moms being upset because their babies were born prematurely at thirty-five weeks. Their tears in the feeding room were annoying because I knew from reading every possible book and website about premature babies that their babies would be just fine. I tried to understand their disappointment but when imagining Oklyn's future development, her story always seemed to be the scariest.

In September, Oklyn was still in the nursery. I knew that she was well on her way home as her due date had been September 17th. She was doing well, but was still little and she tired out easily while feeding. We were now waiting for her to get stronger so she could feed properly at home and continue to gain weight.

It was in early September when Oklyn had her last setback. The nurses discovered that Oklyn had an inguinal hernia. At first, they were able to push it back in, but it became obvious that she would need this hernia repaired. She was going to need surgery down in Voulder at the General Children's Hospital. I could not believe this. We were going to have to fly back to Voulder and Oklyn would have to stay once again in the Voulder General Children's Hospital's NICU, a place where I had vowed never to return. I was devastated with this news! This meant that Oklyn would have to stay in the hospital even longer before she was ready to come home with Mack and me. I remember driving home and asking our protector, whoever it was that saved my life and Oklyn's that June 22nd, to give me the strength to cross one more hurdle. I started to read every possible entry on the Internet related to inguinal hernia. I found out that there was a very low risk of death in repairing a hernia if performed on a five-pound baby. There was no choice in the matter. If her hernia was to erupt, it would be extremely dangerous. So once more we waited for the Infant Transport Team to come get us and we flew off to Voulder for another round.

The morning after our arrival in Voulder, Oklyn underwent a second MRI. The study in which we enrolled her when she was first born consisted of having an MRI done at birth and one around her prescribed due date. Initially, Oklyn would not have been able to have the second MRI done as I had not planned to drive her down to Voulder for this procedure. But since we had to be there for the hernia operation anyway, it was a good opportunity to go through with it. When Oklyn returned from the MRI, she had been fasting for six hours and was very agitated. As I was trying to soothe her in preparation for her surgery, four doctors walked into the room. I recognised the primary neurologist of the study. They had horrible news: the second MRI was showing signs of white matter injury. The result was now abnormal, Oklyn's brain was abnormal. I do not remember anything else from this conversation. I was confused and couldn't understand why her brain had changed. Was it my fault? I was already feeling guilty for not protecting her enough. I thought I caused this brain injury to her while taking care of her. In my mind I started to replay the movie of her life since birth to find out when her brain went from normal to abnormal. I remembered one or two times when she had choked while feeding and receiving her medication. Once she also had had a desaturation because I hadn't been holding her properly. I had so many unanswered questions, but didn't want to ask any as I was afraid to hear what I didn't want to hear. I was afraid to hear that I needed to prepare myself for the extra care, therapy or treatment that Oklyn would need all throughout her life.

A few minutes later, Oklyn was taken to the operating room to have her hernia repaired. Next to this new information, the hernia operation seemed of minor importance. I was devastated about what I had just heard. I left the NICU to call Mack who was still in Everwood working. I didn't know where to start! I didn't know how to break the news. I was sobbing so much while trying to talk to him that he thought Oklyn had died while having her hernia repaired. Mack told me to sit down and to wait for him as he would be there in four hours. I just didn't know how to calm myself anymore. During these endless four hours I reran the movie of her life since birth. I sat there and played it repeatedly. The only answer that I was able to find was that I was the one who had done this to her, I was the guilty one. It made sense for me to think that way because I was the only non-professional giving her care. I had almost killed my baby at birth and now I was guilty for giving her this brain injury. I had failed at being a mom, Oklyn's mom.

When Mack arrived, I was still a mess so he requested a meeting with the study's primary neurologist to try to comprehend what was going on and to discuss the results. I didn't want to attend this meeting. I just wanted to sit in the NICU and cuddle with Oklyn who was back from her surgery and doing well.

Mack came back and told me the same news that I had heard. The MRI had shown signs of white matter injury. What did that mean? Were we talking about a severe handicap? Was Oklyn going to be able to walk, was she going to be able to talk, was she even going to be able to sit properly? Was she going to be in a wheelchair? Again, there were so many unanswered questions. We were told that because it was only a study they could not supply any answers. Their research was to see if there was a relation between those injuries and future developmental problems. I was mad at myself for agreeing to have Oklyn involved in this study. I had thought that we were well on our way home and that I was going to see the end of this nightmare. Now it felt like the nightmare was really just beginning and that in a couple of days we would be home on our own without any nurses around and any doctors on call. It was going to be Mack, me, Oklyn, and her injured brain. That MRI result was erasing all my hope. I was now fearing and dreading the day of Oklyn's discharge. The neurologist told us to enjoy our baby, stimulate her as much as we could, and come back for a follow-up at eighteen months and again at three years old. A day later, the Infant Transport Team came to pick us up and take us to the Everwood Queen's Hospital where she would be officially discharged. It was Oklyn's fourth plane ride and she was not even supposed to be born yet.

When we got back to the Everwood Queen's Hospital's NICU, Oklyn's doctor thought that she was almost ready to go home and that we should all prepare for the transition. In order to go home, Oklyn had to show growth, steadily gain weight, take all her feedings by bottle or breast without supplemental tube feedings and pass a car seat test. Premature babies often do not have the muscle control required to keep their heads upright or to move if they are having trouble breathing. The car seat test consisted of Oklyn being placed in the car seat and being connected to a monitor that would evaluate her heart rate and breathing. To successfully pass the test, Oklyn needed to demonstrate that she could sit in her car seat for ninety minutes without experiencing desaturation or a decrease in her heart rate. I was not ready for her to be discharged, and I was even hoping that Oklyn would fail the test so we could stay at the hospital longer.

Oklyn didn't fail the car seat test. She was now feeding really well by bottle and was steadily gaining weight. She was meeting all the necessary requirements. She could now be discharged. Oklyn was ready for her life at home, but I was not! I was very dependent on the nurses and the monitor. Oklyn had been connected to a monitor since birth, even while she was feeding. The monitor measured her heart and breathing rate, her blood pressure and her blood's supply of oxygen. An alarm would ring if she was choking while feeding or if her airway was not open while I was holding her. With the monitor, I knew when to stop feeding or when to change her position. There were a couple of nurses who had noticed my fear of handling her while she was not connected to the monitor. In order to help me become independent, they started to make me disconnect her every time I visited. At first, I was not even going to the feeding room on my own. There was always a nurse coming with me so I would feel safer. I remember crying and shaking while feeding Oklyn just because I was afraid she'd choke and injure her brain even more. The nurses were patient with me and they gradually taught me to look at my baby's face to see what she was telling me. I had to learn that reading Oklyn's face was more accurate than waiting for an alarm to set off a monitor. I was getting better at it, but I was secretly searching on the Internet to find that very same monitor so that I could get some rest in between her feedings at night. A nurse convinced me that if Oklyn still needed a monitor, she wouldn't be coming home. Unlike me, Mack was ready for Oklyn to come home, and that was giving me the confidence to believe that I actually could handle this. He was not stressed like I was or maybe he was just not showing it at the time, but his calmness was helping me manage my fears.

On September 25th, Oklyn's doctor asked me to room in with Oklyn for a night and do all of her care for a twenty-four hour period. I was happy to do this as I thought it would help build my confidence. Oklyn and I were sent to the paediatric floor on the afternoon of the 25th where a bedroom was waiting for us. It did help to spend the night with her, but it also tired me out before having her come home because I was just not able to close my eyes. I was again lost in my thoughts. All night I thought about losing Oklyn. I had waited for so long for the day when Oklyn could come home, but now that the day was here, I could not make myself celebrate it because my feelings were caught up between joy and worry. I would had loved to call friends and family or e-mail them or visit them to introduce Oklyn. I wanted to announce that Oklyn was going to be with us forever. But I was too afraid that once she came home, I would lose her from one of the many problems that I had seen at the Voulder General Children's Hospital. I had seen so many children suffering from different diseases and had heard so many parents sharing their sad stories during our stay at the hospital that I was now always going to be worried about losing my daughter. During that night I tried to get rid of those feelings, but they returned stronger than ever. I realized then that this joy and worry would always be with me. It would make me become the mom I am today, a mom who, despite my joy, worries all of the time.

On a cloudy afternoon on September 26th, we were finally discharged. After ninety-seven hospitalised days, our five-pound, nine-ounce baby was finally coming home. Following a quick stop in the NICU to thank all the wonderful staff, we were on our way home, Oklyn's new home. We were leaving behind us all the difficulties that Oklyn had overcome in her neonatal period: edema, respiratory distress syndrome/hyaline membrane, apnea of prematurity, chronic lung disease, patent ductus arteriosus, hypotension, hernia repaired, jaundice and a change in her white brain matter. We were feeling relieved to leave all of this behind us, but we were also feeling anxious because we didn't know what was coming next and what new difficulties we could encounter. Was bringing a premature baby home different than bringing a full-term baby home? We were leaving the Everwood Queen's Hospital without saying or hearing one single word about what had been found on the second MRI. I wanted to leave that story at Voulder General Children's Hospital and never hear about it again.

I would be lying if I said that Oklyn's arrival home was smooth and that it brought the comfort I had been craving since the beginning of this adventure. I would also be lying if I said that her first couple of months at home were fun. There was a constant stress in our home. We had done and bought everything possible to keep Oklyn safe, but it was still not enough to give us peace of mind, especially at night. Mack and I were on "baby care shifts" so there was always someone awake in our house. Oklyn was a very bad sleeper. She would only sleep while on her stomach and because we had read so much about Sudden Infant Death Syndrome (SIDS) and how babies should not sleep on their stomachs, we felt we had to watch her all the time if that was how she was sleeping. We could never close our eyes. I remember reading that SIDS was most common with babies aged between two to four months, so I spent these months crossing the days off the calendar. When Oklyn reached four months, I started to worry about her not "babbling" and so again I started to cross off days on the calendar, but this time I wanted to go backwards. I didn't want her to reach that date, the day that babies are supposed to babble according to "Dr. So-and-So" on the Internet. I became obsessed with the Internet during Oklyn's first year of life. I was always researching about prematurity and about infant milestones. The doctors warned us not to go online to research what we had heard in the NICU. They told us to go to them instead, but we were hearing so many new words that it was making it impossible to stay away from the world wide web. Not only were doctors introducing new words to us, but everywhere we went we were surrounded by people who were going through tough times with their premature babies or who knew of others who were going through a similar experience. The Internet became a useful tool, but also a very devastating one. I found relief and comfort in some stories that I read, but it also initiated fears. There was always a tension in our home that I was just not able to control.

My maternity leave was quite different from the ones that my friends were experiencing. My friends were having play dates, lunches out with their babies and even going to movies for parents with babies. My days were spent at home or around the neighbourhood walking Oklyn to help her fall asleep. We never took her anywhere near a friend's house, a store or a restaurant because we were so afraid that she would get sick. I was also afraid that Oklyn did not have the muscle control required to keep her head upright or to adjust it if she was having trouble breathing in the car seat. Consequently, I never drove anywhere with her. My days were boring and depressing. I was starting to feel trapped. I needed an escape, but that was not possible as Mack was working five days a week from 8:30 am to 6:30 pm. Furthermore, I was afraid to entrust anyone else with my little Oklyn. I was not going to leave my precious baby after all the hard work she had done to stay alive. I was obviously becoming this crazy mom, the mom who worries all of the time.

Oklyn's first months with us were monitored closely by

nurses who would come to our home. Oklyn's progress was followed weekly for her weight and monthly for her development in other areas. She was also seeing a physiotherapist and a paediatrician. Being Oklyn's mom was now my full-time job. I remember enjoying the nurses' visits as I would get to spend some time with an adult and to interact with someone else besides Mack. New parents often find these visits overwhelming, but for me it was a chance to do something else besides obsess about Oklyn's future.

Even though we were doing everything possible to keep Oklyn away from germs, she was still experiencing setbacks that were not in our power to control. After finding blood in Oklyn's stool, we discovered she was severely lactose intolerant and needed to be put on a special formula. I even put myself on a special diet so that I could still feed her with my breast milk without giving her stomach pain. During this time, Oklyn also got a couple of urinary tract infections that sent her back to the hospital for a few days, the time needed for the antibiotics to kill the infections. These trips to Oklyn's doctor and her sojourns in the hospital would have been devastating for many new parents, but for Mack and me it was almost something we expected. I was still feeling very fragile, but I was starting to have a shell that was protecting me from Oklyn's setbacks and protecting me from being discouraged. I needed to keep going. I needed to stay strong to care for a baby who needed a mentally healthy mom, so again I brushed all my feelings aside and concentrated on the most important thing - taking care of Oklyn.

Things started to improve when I decided to stop breastfeeding Oklyn and concentrate only on pumping my milk for her bottle. Oklyn's sucking was still not strong enough to allow her to be feed by breast alone. Consequently, feeding Oklyn was a very long task as I was first breastfeeding her, then pumping my remaining milk afterwards. I would then use this pumped milk to top her up. Feeding her was sometimes taking more than an hour and half, and I would often have to start all over an hour later. I decided that for the duration of a year, rather than directly breastfeed, I would pump and then bottle feed her with my breast milk. After that decision, my life began to be easier and it gave me more time to focus on Oklyn. The two of us developed our own daily routine. I would massage her for an hour every day, give her a long bath and take her outside for a walk in the morning and the afternoon. Oklyn was acting like every other baby; she was smiling, she seemed content and she was starting to hold up her neck. This allowed the two of us to go for car rides. Finally, we were able to walk somewhere else besides our own neighbourhood. I was now able to sit in the front seat of the car when Mack was driving, but Oklyn was still not going to friends' houses, stores or restaurants.

Oklyn's progress continued to be followed by the Infant Development Program (IDP) and she was assessed by the consultant on each visit. Our consultant reported that Oklyn was doing very well. The assessment was not showing anything wrong with her. I was starting to believe that Oklyn was going to be able to sit, walk, play and be just like any other little girl.

In early November, while we were having one of our regular paediatrician's visit, I summoned the courage to mention the MRI's findings. This paediatician had been there with us since the beginning and I wanted to know her opinion about the brain injury found on Oklyn's second MRI. To my surprise, she hadn't known anything about this and was not very happy to hear that we had been told to go home and wait to see. She is an amazing doctor who really has her patients' best interests at heart. She called the primary neurologist for the study to discuss the results of the MRI. As I was holding Oklyn and trying to keep her quiet so our doctor could talk to the neurologist, I started to smile and smile and smile as I listened to their conversation. I was overjoyed to hear them say that the MRI result apparently showed nothing major, and that it could perhaps end up that Oklyn might develop nothing more threatening than a minor attention deficit hyperactivity disorder. I could not believe it! I was elated, but also angry. I had spent the last two months feeling guilty, having nightmares and obsessing all day about what Oklyn's future might entail. Now I was finally losing this extra burden that I had been carrying on my shoulders since the day I was told the devastating MRI news. I was angry and upset with this study, but I was not going to waste my energy dwelling on the negative aspects because I was just so happy to be able to smile and feel so relieved again. I was now certain that I was not guilty and that I hadn't failed at being Oklyn's mom. Was I going to be able to finally find the peace I was looking for since Oklyn's delivery?

That Christmas, December 2008, my parents came to visit us. It was not their first visit with Oklyn. They had flown to Voulder when she was first born. This time they thought that Oklyn was still very little, but not as fragile as I had been describing her over the phone. They were happy to see that she was developing just like any other little girl, but were sad to see that I was not treating her that way. I was still treating Oklyn like a premature and fragile baby. My mom thought I needed to hear what she had to say. She made me realise that Oklyn was not the one who was fragile anymore, but that it was me. She made me understand that I had done everything in my power to keep Oklyn safe and that it was time for me to consider my daughter as a four month old and that she was growing just fine. It was not a pleasant conversation, but it was a very truthful one. I needed to hear what she had to say and seriously consider her advice for my own mental health, and I did! Over the month of January, I gradually started to introduce Oklyn to the outside world. We visited public places to try to experience a little bit more normalcy. After a couple of weeks living a more normal life, I realised that Oklyn was not sick and that she was developing as well as when she was locked up at home, possibly even better. In February, Oklyn went with us to Santa Barbara, California for her first pleasure trip. Two weeks later, I took Oklyn to Quebec for her second holiday. On our way back from our Quebec trip, I had a revealing moment! I came to the conclusion that in order to develop normally, Oklyn needed to be exposed to the world. However Oklyn's development would fare in the future, it would never change my love for her. Oklyn was my daughter and I was so proud of her. During that plane ride I also realised that we were going to be fine and that I needed to give Oklyn the space she needed to develop and evolve as her own person. I needed to back off!

After almost a year, I was able to sit down and not always be lost in my negative thoughts. I was able to smile, laugh and celebrate each milestone that Oklyn was reaching and not dwell on her not making it to the next one. It was now comforting to put Oklyn to bed at night and find the peace and solace that Mack and I were looking for and deserved after such a long and arduous journey.

Let's Do This Again!

As mothers we seem to forget very quickly the delivery pain, the tiring sleepless nights and the inconsolable cries that our little angels make when they become part of our world. Personally, I cannot really say what exactly drove me to make an appointment with an obstetrician nine months after delivering Oklyn. I certainly wanted two children. There was no doubt in my mind that two little angels were going to be better than just one in my house. But before making it happen, I needed to know if it was even feasible, considering what had happened with my first pregnancy. I just knew I was not capable of repeating the "Oklyn experience" twice in my life. To this day, there is still something inexplicable that was driving me to have another child. I remember reading online that 95% of women who had experienced a premature delivery for their first child wanted to get pregnant again in the next eighteen months.

I felt I had been robbed with Oklyn's pregnancy because I just hadn't had the opportunity to experience the pleasure of being pregnant for the complete nine months. I felt that I had missed out on many things when the HELLP syndrome robbed me of the perfect pregnancy I had dreamed of. I simply wanted to have a full-term baby, a big round belly, a stress-free maternity leave and the pleasure of raising two children just the way I had been brought up. This time I wanted to prove that I could carry the baby full term and that it had just been bad luck with Oklyn. My first pregnancy had left me disappointed in myself, but this pregnancy would prove that I could do it right. I just wanted to have a healthy baby and I was positive that I could achieve this goal. I was healthy, the blood tests ordered by the obstetrician were normal, there was no trace of distress on my kidneys and liver from the first pregnancy. I was given the green light by my obstetrician, but he did say that I would need to be closely monitored.

Mack and I had not been discussing having another baby. We were already very busy with Oklyn. She was only nine months old, really just six months "corrected." Correcting her age is something that we were taught to do for her development. It would have been unfair to consider Oklyn as a three-month-old when she was discharged from the hospital. When doctors wanted to know if she was reaching the developmental milestones, they used the date on which she was supposed to be born. It was sometimes confusing for people when they asked us how old Oklyn was as I often used the corrected age and Mack used her birth age. People would often ask us what was her real age and I just answered, "That it is a good question!"

The doctor informed me that there was a 4% chance for

the HELLP syndrome to reoccur if we got pregnant for a second time. This made Mack hesitant to have another baby. I told him that I really wanted to have another one and that we could wait until the summer to make the final decision. I think he was more afraid than I was because he had seen more than I had during the minutes before and after Oklyn's delivery. Having another baby was not part of our everyday conversation until Mother's Day. On that day, Mack gave me a beautiful card, and in it he had written a wonderful message declaring that he wanted me to be a mother for a second time. I was happy to read that he wanted another child just like I did, but I still was not totally ready to go there. First, I wanted to make sure that Oklyn was truly developing normally.

When July came, we decided to try having a second baby. We thought that it had taken us almost a year to conceive Oklyn, so we could start trying and hope for the best. This time we didn't get to practice as much because a few weeks later I found out that I was pregnant! I could not believe that it had worked that quickly. Just like the statistics had predicted, I got pregnant just a little after Oklyn celebrated her first uncorrected year. I was thrilled, but I was also haunted by some scary thoughts.

I thought that this time it was different right from the start. I was vomiting numerous times a day and was exhausted. The doctor said that it was good news as it meant my placenta was working well. The first few months were uneventful. I was keeping myself busy with being back at work full time and taking care of a one-year-old. I made the big announcement to my friends and teaching staff around the eleventh week of the pregnancy and to my surprise, people around me seemed excited for us. I had thought people would question our decision about having another baby as we hadn't really talked about another addition. But they sounded happy that Oklyn was going to have a brother or a sister.

The doctors had advised me that I would not be monitored closely until around the twenty-second week, when the fetus would be considered "viable" which means capable of surviving outside the womb with artificial support. It was around the fourteenth week that this pregnancy went from being moderately stressful to very worrisome. I was having a routine prenatal visit with my doctor where a simple physical exam was going to be done. After many attempts, the doctor couldn't find the heartbeat so he immediately sent me to see an obstetrician in the delivery room. Fortunately, just like the first time, an obstetrician from the Voulder General Hospital happened to be visiting Everwood Queen's Hospital. She was able to find the heartbeat quickly, but it was the following conversation that got my attention. After I gave her a little update about my first pregnancy she recommended that I see a specialist at the Voulder General Hospital who would order a Uterine Artery Doppler test to see how the blood flow was going between myself and the baby. The pictures would show the specialist how well the placenta was developing and how effectively it was likely to do its job for the rest of the pregnancy. My doctor thought that I would not want to drive to Voulder General Hospital to have this test done, but it was just the opposite: I wanted to see every possible specialist in order to avoid having a repeat of my first pregnancy. I must have made myself clearly heard because that same day a referral was sent to the Voulder General Hospital.

Two long, stressful weeks later I had an appointment with an obstetrician-gynaecologist who was currently the President of the North American Society for the Study of Hypertension in Pregnancy. The title in itself was scaring me. I was expected to be at the hospital at 7:30am for a Uterine Artery Doppler test, an ultrasound, a physical exam with a nurse and a consultation with the specialist. My visit to the hospital would last over three hours. I made my way there alone. Although Mack and Oklyn had accompanied me to Voulder, we felt that they should wait for me back at the condo. We both thought that Oklyn would be overwhelmed by a three-hour appointment at the hospital. I was already stressed and nervous when I parked my car. It felt so much like déjà vu. The staff at the Voulder General Hospital was just as courteous as I had remembered them, but I was too preoccupied to enjoy their polite greetings. There was a voice inside of me saying that I had not been sent here for good news, so while waiting to see the specialist I could not help but be extremely worried. Seeing other pregnant women in the waiting room was not helping me as they were all in their third trimester and I was only at the beginning of my second. So why was I here so early in this pregnancy? Was I going to be their worst case that day? Reading this, you may wonder why I felt so worried. After all, the doctors had only sent me here as a precaution. But you have to realize that for me there was always something to worry about.

The appointment with the nurse went well. All I had to do was answer the usual questions that any pregnant woman would answer at a first prenatal visit. I was uncomfortable though, when a student intern was sent to ask me questions related to my first pregnancy. His pointed questions were really taking me back to my first experience. Believe it or not, this was the first time that I had spoken to someone so intimately and shared my deepest, most innermost thoughts. He wanted to know everything from beginning to end. I was already getting a little sensitive about it and we were only talking about the past and not at all about what was ahead of me for this second pregnancy. His questions were taking me back to the first pregnancy, and I was beginning to worry that there was a chance I would have to go through that nightmare pregnancy all over again.

Then I was introduced to the specialist. His accent reminded me of the doctors I saw the night that I delivered Oklyn. He was from New Zealand and appeared to be self-confident, funny and understanding. However, he didn't have good news for me. There was already a 60% chance that I was going to deliver a premature baby. To him it was nothing surprising. In fact, he wondered why I was surprised. He told me that the HELLP syndrome does reoccur in a second pregnancy in almost every case and that women who have already suffered from it should wait at least two years before getting pregnant again. He was surprised that the Everwood Queen's Hospital obstetrician had not warned me of this. Why wasn't I told about this when I consulted the specialist in Everwood? I got very upset because I was positive that if I had known what he was telling me before conceiving, I would not be having another baby. But what could I do now? I was already pregnant. He assured me that there were also good things going on. By this, he meant that the HELLP syndrome would reoccur later during this pregnancy than it had during the first, and that it would not be as aggressive. But his words were falling on deaf ears. I was not listening to him anymore. I was already lost in my thoughts, disturbing as they were, because I had been there before. As the appointment progressed, I became more and more anxious. There was talk about relocating to Voulder to deliver at the General Hospital and have the baby wheeled down the hall to the General Children's Hospital. This would provide for the best start for the baby in the best place in the entire province. I was even told that Oklyn had saved my life because women who suffer from the HELLP syndrome have a greater risk of suffering from heart disease in the future. Without having children, I would not have known that I was at risk. I left the hospital with a note telling my employer that I needed to be off work as soon as possible and with another appointment scheduled in two weeks time.

After breaking the news to Mack we were on our way home to Everwood, both of us shedding many tears along the way. We were so confused and disappointed. The next two weeks were busy. I had to give my notice at work, hastily complete report cards and tie up loose ends. We told our family, friends and co-workers our latest news, and they all gave us their support and nod of approval. It was interesting, though, to hear some of their reactions, as it caused me to wonder if all the congratulations they had given us the previous months had been entirely honest. I was questioned about our choice of wanting another baby after having gone through so much with Oklyn. I felt judged and misunderstood. Reading between the lines of their remarks, it really did sound to me like they thought that I was being selfish for wanting another baby, or that I hadn't used my common sense before conceiving, and that I was being greedy for taking such a risk. Accurate or not, these comments at this time were hurtful and not helping me.

Two weeks later we were back at Voulder General Hospital for my second appointment. This time Mack joined me. We agreed that he needed to be there so that we could both hear and better understand what the doctor had to tell us. I needed someone strong beside me to ask the important questions when I would began to feel overwhelmed with what the future might hold for us. After going through a Uterine Artery Doppler and an ultrasound again, we were sent to the doctor's office. Mack and I were both prepared with a list of questions. The news was not good. In fact, it was even worse than what we'd heard after the first appointment. The chance of my delivering a premature baby had increased from 60% to 80%, my blood pressure was already elevated and the fetus had dropped from the fiftieth to the eleventh percentile on the growth chart. Due to my placenta not working properly, the baby was already showing signs of growth restrictions. I was not even twenty weeks pregnant.

We certainly had numerous troubling questions to ask the doctor. When was this baby going to be born? Was there a chance that I could die from this? How small would the baby be if its growth was already restricted? And the biggest question of all: should we end this pregnancy? Mack and I believe in pro-choice, which is to give women the choice of whether or not to get an abortion. But this is not an easy decision and we wanted the doctor's opinion as well. It turned out that he was pro-choice too! We wanted and needed to have an honest opinion of what to do. I remember asking him what he would recommend to his daughter if she was in a similar situation. Mack and I were confused and upset, but we were clear about what we wanted or didn't want. We didn't want a baby born before twenty-seven weeks, as Oklyn had been, because we were too afraid of what the outcome would be. We were already feeling so lucky that Oklyn was developing just fine and didn't want to push our luck any further.

The doctor did have an opinion for us! He thought we needed to wait before making a final decision. He wanted to see us again in two weeks to undergo the same testing and see if the fetus was going to stay in the eleventh percentile or drop again. If the placenta growth was still around the eleventh percentile, his advice was that we should continue with the pregnancy. This didn't completely satisfy us. We were still not positive about waiting because we thought that as difficult as it would be to end the pregnancy now, it would be even more difficult to end it in two weeks time if the results were again unfavourable. The doctor made us talk about our fears of having a baby before the twenty-seventh week. We all agreed to not resuscitate the baby if it was born before the twenty-fifth week. We were also afraid of a low birth weight baby. Babies born under five hundred grams were usually not resuscitated, but we wanted to make sure that the growth restriction was not going to make me deliver a lower-weight baby than Oklyn's eight hundred and forty grams. Low weight babies can often have many complications. The doctor then said something that made both Mack and me sit up. He suggested that I take Viagra! We wondered if we had heard him correctly. It sounded weird until he explained that taking Viagra would increase the uterine blood flow and that it is well known to doctors that a restriction of uterine blood flow during pregnancy is associated with growth restriction of the fetus. If I took Viagra, the fetus would grow normally for a couple of weeks, then it would stop again. The doctor wanted Mack and me to discuss this over the next weeks and make a decision regarding taking the medication or not. Mack and I knew that there was a risk for my life and the baby's as well, and we wanted to know if I would be closely monitored. The doctor replied that the mothers were taken care of and yes, I would be well monitored. Then he started to educate us. He explained that if I aborted, I would carry guilt and regret for the rest of my life. He wanted me to understand that it would be a very long grief. People around me would not understand my feelings. I would need to see a psychiatrist. As a teacher, I would have to face children all day long and it would be a constant reminder of my lost baby. I wondered if he was pro-life more than pro-choice. But we had his support no matter what decision we opted to choose, and he would also help us with all the arrangements if ending the pregnancy was going to be our choice. Mack and I liked him and we were confident that he had a good understanding of the disease, but we were also feeling like one of his experiments, as there are so many studies around this illness. On our way out, we again made another appointment to return within the next two weeks to undergo the testing once more.

Our family and friends generously offered their opinions, many recommending pro-life and as many voting for pro-choice. The pro-choicers were thinking about my health and about the fact that I was now a mom of a healthy little girl who, more than anything else, just needed a healthy mother. I could sense that they didn't want the responsibility to tell me to end the pregnancy, but it is really what they were hoping for. At the same time, the pro-lifers were making me feel guilty for wanting another child a couple of months ago and now not being sure if we should abort because of the unexpected bad news we were receiving. They were making me feel irresponsible and cold-hearted. The doctor was right on when he said people would not understand our decision. I wanted, and expected, family and friends to give me their opinion, but after a while I was starting to get annoyed with being told what to do.

I was deeply troubled. I often felt that we already had one miracle and that we would not be lucky again and have another healthy baby. Mack took the opposite approach. He said that we had had our rough time, and that this one was going to be easier. But I knew that he wasn't that sure about all of this. He had thought that he was going to lose both of us during the first delivery. I think that deep down it scared him enough to want to make sure we would never go through this again. We were avoiding talking about it.

We were waiting for the third appointment before making a decision. We agreed that if the baby stopped growing, there was no point continuing the pregnancy. Having a preemie was a huge challenge, but having an underweight preemie was going to be a catastrophe, and we were not willing to go there.

I totally trusted the specialist at Voulder General Hospital, but still wanted a second opinion so I continued to see the obstetrician at Everwood Queen's Hospital. He was aware of my circumstances, as he was receiving the reports from the General Hospital. I was very curious about his opinion. To my surprise, he didn't seem to believe that there was much of a problem. He was not prepared to allow numbers to play a major role in this pregnancy. When I talked to him about ending the pregnancy if the fetus wasn't growing, he didn't understand where I was coming from. He asked me if I really wanted to have this baby in first place, to be making such a radical decision. I thought he was not listening to me and was not giving me the second opinion I was searching for. When I left his office, I told myself that I needed to seriously think about relocating to Voulder for the duration of this pregnancy as I was not going to find the professional help I was looking for in Everwood.

The two-week period between appointments was dragging on, and every passing day was making me more anxious. I didn't want to end this pregnancy. I wanted to have another child, and furthermore, I didn't feel strong enough to go through an abortion. I knew an abortion would be excruciatingly painful emotionally and it would take months, and even years, for me to move on. I thought for sure that I would become a woman who would cry every time babies were brought up in conversations. Friends and family would have to be painstakingly patient with me to help me move on and not be regretful for the rest of my life. However, having this baby was going to be a real challenge also. Giving birth to a premature baby wasn't going to be a smooth ride. Was the baby going to be healthy? How long was the baby going to be at the hospital? Oklyn was now with us and needed my care as much as a new baby. When would I go visit the new arrival at the hospital? I could certainly not spend my days staring at my new baby in the incubator like I did with Oklyn. Would I be able to pump for a whole year while having Oklyn at home with me? I was lost in my thoughts even more than ever and could not be comforted. I just had to wait and wait and wait for the third appointment.

Our third appointment at the Voulder General Hospital finally arrived and, for the first time since meeting this doctor, he had good news for us. The fetus was still growing and was now between the tenth and twentieth percentile on the growth chart. We were going to keep this baby! We were also told that we were expecting another baby girl. We were so happy to hear this because we had been told many times with Oklyn that premature girls fare better than premature boys. I felt somewhat relieved but not totally, as I was still going to deliver a premature baby and was not yet twenty-four weeks pregnant. I remember Mack telling me to focus on the good news and not dwell on what could happen in the future. He always sounded positive, and it was helping me to keep it together. After that appointment we also decided that we would relocate to Voulder to the condo where we stayed when Oklyn was born. I felt, though, like the doctor was rushing us to come and live in Voulder and I didn't understand why. We were clear on not resuscitating the baby if born before twenty-five weeks so why did we need to relocate so soon? Was he not telling us the truth? Were the tests showing something we were not aware of? Where did the actual concern lie?

Christmas time arrived and we were told by the doctor to enjoy the holidays. Both our families were only a plane ride away but I was not allowed to fly in this condition so we ended up celebrating Christmas with friends in Everwood. I remember asking for only one present over the holidays - for my mom to be healthy enough to come and help us once we moved to Voulder. In order to be able to leave Oklyn for an undetermined amount of time when I was hospitalized, I needed someone with whom I would feel comfortable to look after her.

I was relieved that my mom was eager to come and help us out. After spending Christmas and New Year's Day in Everwood, we moved to Voulder. I was not looking forward to our life there since I was going through a high-risk pregnancy with no one around to support me. Of course there was Mack, but he was very busy with work and my mom wouldn't be joining us for another two weeks. It was difficult for Oklyn and me to adjust, as Voulder was just not home. We were both used to play dates with friends and a big house where she was able to run around. However, I was happy to do this so that my baby girl would get the best possible start to her life. I was already in love with this baby who was staying so strong inside of my belly.

Very quickly after Christmas I went from seeing the doctor every second week to seeing him weekly. I was also introduced to another doctor whom I would see once a week to monitor my blood pressure. I was now being cared for by two specialists – one was taking care of the baby, watching what the ultrasound was showing, and the other was taking care of my health, as my blood pressure was starting to escalate again.

My mom was now with us and it was making our lives so much easier. Oklyn was able to stay at home with her when I was going to the hospital. Between all the appointments and caring for Oklyn at home, I was very busy. It was a difficult situation for me but was also a good opportunity for my mom, Oklyn and me to spend quality time together. My mom lived far away, so it was good for Oklyn to be able to reconnect with her "Mamie" again. Living in a small condo and adjusting to big city Voulder was difficult for all of us but we were trying to make the best of it. Between my appointments, we were enjoying walks on the beach and play dates with some other children from the community. I didn't want Oklyn to be deprived just because we were going through a difficult time. I was praying every day that Oklyn's sister would be as healthy and as strong as Oklyn was.

Mack and I were keeping our fingers crossed that I would not deliver until my pregnancy moved along to twenty-seven weeks and four days. Oklyn had survived at that age, and so, we hoped, would our new little girl. I was becoming very anxious as this date was fast approaching, and yet it wasn't coming soon enough. I was now spending most of my nights on the couch worrying. Sometimes I was barely sleeping. The thought of giving birth to another premature baby was very scary and was keeping me awake. I remember spending nights playing with my wedding ring and wondering if it felt smaller than the day before, because swollen fingers are a sign of preeclampsia. I was also weighing myself every morning on a digital scale to see exactly how much I was gaining, as a fast weight gain means water retention, another sign of preeclampsia. The disease was controlling my mind, and as the days were trickling by, I was becoming more and more obsessed with the fear of delivering a premature baby. I had no patience for Oklyn or my mom because my thoughts were focused solely on delivering my baby later than twenty-seven weeks and four days.

The twenty-seven weeks and four days gestational age came on a Monday, the same day that I was having an ultrasound and a consultation with the doctor. That day, the doctor didn't have good news. The baby was no longer growing, and I needed medication for my blood pressure as it was too elevated. He also told me that I would need to sit on the couch as much as possible, to help add more weeks to this pregnancy. It was great to have my mom around so that Oklyn could still do some fun things. It would have been too complicated for a sixteen-month-old little girl to understand why her mom couldn't move around much anymore.

The growth restriction changed the routine I had for my

appointments. The new plan was to have an ultrasound and a blood pressure check twice a week. The baby's heart rate needed to be monitored every second day. I knew this routine would be short-lived, as I was having the same symptoms that I had had just before delivering Oklyn. I was gaining about one pound a day, my urine smelled different, my ankles were swollen and I had little white spots all over my legs. I talked to the doctor about all of these changes but he kept telling me that everything was fine. My blood tests were still normal and the ultrasound showed a healthy baby. There was no doubt in my mind that all of my problems were pointing towards an early delivery. I was now spending my nights sitting up awake because I was too afraid to die in my sleep. My blood pressure was still very high, even on medication, and I was not feeling well at all.

It was on a Thursday that my symptoms finally caught the attention of a nurse. I was in the hospital having the baby's heart rate monitored, and the baby wasn't moving and kicking enough. She was just not giving us the results we wanted so the nurse suggested that I see a doctor. The doctor thought I should be admitted for one night to make sure things were all right. I knew that my baby girl was starting to suffer too much and that she needed to be delivered. I told the doctor that I had been in this same situation once before and I knew the delivery was just a matter of hours away. She laughed and told me to calm down and stay positive, as my admission was simply a cautionary routine check. I was sent to a bedroom upstairs at the Voulder General Hospital where I was told to rest until the doctor would come to assess the situation. I was not feeling too bad except that I was suffering from a very painful headache situated in the back of my head. It was almost like a neck ache. Throughout that afternoon my blood samples were taken and the results all came back normal. But the headache became more violent as the afternoon wore on, and I complained about it. The nurse told me that it was probably caused by stress and by being hungry and dehydrated, as my schedule had changed quite a bit that day. What she said made sense but deep down I recognized all the symptoms, and they really were not caused by a sudden change in my schedule. I spent that afternoon thinking about the next step and being angry because this was happening again to me, to us. I was even angrier when I saw some of the other pregnant women on the ward who were smoking, obese or in their fifties. There was an Asian woman beside my bedroom who was fifty-two years old and expecting twins. It just wasn't fair to me, to us!

The doctor arrived at 6:00 pm and she soon diagnosed me with preeclampsia. My blood pressure was more elevated, medication was not easing my headache, and my reflexes were hyperactive. Only six hours after being admitted, I was sent to the Emergency ward to be closely monitored. After numerous tests, I was told that my blood reading was still normal and I didn't need an immediate c-section. Although I was showing symptoms of preeclampsia, my life was not being threatened. I still had an excruciating headache, one like I'd never had before, yet I was told not to worry. Mack spent the night in the room with me because we both knew that this weird unusual headache was a strong clear sign of an early delivery.

Around 5:00 a.m. Mack left to get ready for a busy work day. An hour later, I called to tell him that the results of the latest blood tests were abnormal, and I needed an emergency c-section. I was once again a victim of "Hemolysis, Elevated Liver Enzymes and Low Platelets Syndrome". Do these words sound familiar to you? I was diagnosed with HELLP syndrome.

What came next felt like déjà vu. The parade began! One after another, various doctors were sent in. The obstetrician came first followed by a paediatrician and then the anaesthesist. I don't remember much from their conversations, but I know that both Mack and I didn't feel the need to have all these explanations repeated again. I was twenty-eight weeks pregnant, so we knew what was coming next and we knew all the problems that a baby this early was going to experience. I also remember the nurses arguing about how many bags of platelets I would need for a platelet transfusion. At that moment, I felt very angry because no one had listened to my concerns during the last twenty-four hours and if they had listened, they would know the number of bags needed. They'd be ready! I had had all of the symptoms for an early delivery for more than twenty-four hours and no one had listened.

Koraly was born January 29th at 9:40am. I carried her for twenty-eight weeks to the day and she weighed one pound, fifteen ounces. The doctor was correct when he said that the HELLP syndrome would reoccur a little later in this pregnancy than it had in the first, but I am not sure if can say that the disease was less aggressive. Even though it was happening, I hadn't expected things to escalate that quickly.

There is no need to describe what happened over the next few days. Mack said it all in an e-mail to announce Koraly's birth "Second birth, same as the first". Here is the message that was sent by Mack and me, twenty-four hours after the birth of Koraly.

Hello all. So, we have another little girl. And, not to be outdone by her sister, she arrived before her due date. The sibling rivalry has already started. Oklyn may have come out sooner but Koraly was able to pack on a few more grams than her big sister. She was delivered on January 29th at 9:40 am after preeclampsia reared its ugly head again. Koraly was on a ventilator for most of the day yesterday as a precaution but they removed it as her lungs proved quite strong. At rounds this morning, she was the easiest of the bunch as her stats are great, and all she wants to do is sleep and grow. Melanie has now been moved to the Arbutus ward of Voulder General Hospital and is feeling better. Still a little weary, but she is on the road to recovery. Oklyn is working on her French with her Mamie, and her grampa David has jumped in for some babysitting time. As for the pronunciation of our little girl's name, KO-RA-LY, say it fast and in a French accent. It really sounds quite nice. Good luck to you all and me too. We will update you all when possible.
Mélanie, Mack, Oklyn & Koraly

Reading this e-mail now shows how we were more positive with Koraly's birth, compared to Oklyn's. There were good things going on, as Koraly had a stronger start. No resuscitation was needed, she was born in the best hospital in the province, she was taken care of by specialists very familiar with preemies, and she was expected both by us and the hospital. There were no surprises for us as we always knew what was coming after each step and there were no worried looks exchanged by doctors. However, the concern for us was that she was just twenty-eight weeks and very little. Even though she had had a better start, she was only two ounces bigger than Oklyn had been and only a couple of days older than her sister at delivery. While she was doing better, the difference between the two was minimal. I was familiar with the NICU, but I was still not looking forward to our first introduction as I knew that Koraly would be connected to monitors from head to toe, and that she would be the size of my hand. I was able to visit Koraly sooner than when I had Oklyn, but I felt the same pain. I was introduced to her about twenty-four hours after delivery. This time there was even a new disturbing feeling when I first saw her. It was guilt. I felt sorry for doing this to her. I felt sorry for giving birth to such a tiny baby who would have to fight for her life for at least the first three months.

My hospital stay was much the same as it had been during Oklyn's delivery. The staff who were taking care of Koraly and me were amazing and, to my surprise, some of them recognized us. I stayed at the hospital for seven days, and leaving Koraly the day of my discharge was as painful as when I had left Oklyn but this time I was at least aware of the routine that was to follow.

We were again approached by the same researchers but of all the possible studies, only the MRI study interested me. Honestly, I was not looking forward to having it done, but I knew it was important because it could give us a clear picture of what was going on in Koraly's brain, and help us give her the best possible start. I signed her up for the MRI two days after her delivery. First she had a head ultrasound done and the result came back normal. Then came the MRI. I remember being very angry that they would not share the MRI results over the phone. I felt angry, but I think it was also fear, fear of hearing that her brain was abnormal. Mack finally got in touch with the neurologist and told him that he was causing us great anxiety by not giving us the results. The specialist told him not to worry, as her brain looked normal. I was relieved and I finally did believe that she only needed to eat, sleep and grow.

Koraly's stay at the Voulder General Hospital lasted twenty-nine days. It was a difficult month for me as I had a little girl full of energy at home and one fighting for her life at the hospital. I was constantly feeling guilty as no matter how much loving care I was giving to one daughter, I always had to leave the other one behind. It felt hectic to be at home because Oklyn could not understand why her mom was so busy with everything else besides her. I was pumping eight times a day and going to the hospital two to three times a day so there was not much time for a sixteen-month-old little one who just wanted to play and be loved. It was stressful being at the hospital as I never knew what was coming next. I was now wearing the Supermom cape all day long. But I wasn't sure that it fit me quite right!

Koraly was doing well, much better than Oklyn had done at that age. I could see that expecting her and delivering her at the Voulder General Hospital had been advantageous for Koraly. I had had time to get two shots of steroids before her delivery. The steroids are a benefit for lung development as they reduce the risk of respiratory distress syndrome (RDS) and intracranial hemorrhaging. Koraly was reaching milestones quickly and her daily weight gain was constant. Only fifteen days after delivery, she was breathing on her own and her colors were always good. When the doctor called her "the little star" I'd smile, as I was so proud of my precious little daughter Koraly.

Koraly's stay in the NICU at the Voulder General Children's Hospital was a good opportunity for us to take Oklyn for her eighteen-month follow-up MRI study. Although she was still not eighteen months "corrected," the doctors agreed that it would be fine, and it would make our lives easier if we didn't have to return to Voulder once we had transferred back to Everwood Queen's Hospital. Because of the many professionals involved, the follow-up to the MRI lasted four hours. We met with a physiotherapist, a paediatrician and a neurologist. Oklyn was doing fantastically well and they were very pleased with her development. I truly didn't need their opinion. I knew that Oklyn was doing just fine. I was a little concerned about her language development, but not worried enough to take action. The most interesting part of the meeting was when we all talked about her second MRI. I was told that what they'd seen probably didn't mean much because they were now wondering if the MRI was giving too many details. What I understood was that the images they were getting of her brain were different than the images of a normal brain. The different details seen in her white matter were most likely not going to affect her development. I was again relieved with the news, but also angry. I had spent days and nights worrying about Oklyn's future after the result of that MRI and had to wait sixteen long months to be told that "it was nothing to worry about." I was still upset with the manner in which the neurologist had delivered the results of Oklyn's second MRI, but these results lost their importance to me as I was witnessing with my own eyes that Oklyn was able to cope as well as any of our friends' sixteen-month-old children.

On the 29th day of Koraly's life she was transferred to Everwood Queen's Hospital, as she was healthy and strong. I looked forward to that day because I knew almost everyone in the Everwood Queen's Hospital's nursery and I knew that Koraly would get a great quality of care equal to Oklyn's.

This time my mom flew with Koraly and the Infant Transport Team and I drove with Oklyn. It was such an exciting drive. I knew that all of the stress was coming to an end. I was not going to have another baby, so I could say my farewell to the NICU of the Voulder General Children's Hospital. Koraly was leaving Voulder healthy, with a normal head ultrasound and a normal MRI. After four long months, I was finally able to begin the de-stressing process.

I was comforted that the Everwood Queen's Hospital's

NICU was expecting us and that they were looking forward to taking care of Koraly. It felt like I'd never left the nursery between having Oklyn and then having Koraly. The staff hadn't changed much so it was nice to be able to catch up with everyone. It was also comforting to chat about personal things, not just medical issues. The way they cared for babies was helping me cope with the stress of dealing with a premature baby. However, because I was "experienced," the staff sometimes expected that I already knew everything and didn't need them to explain what was going on. This was difficult for me.

Babies who are born less or equal to 1250 grams get tested for retinopathy of prematurity (ROP). ROP is a disease that affects the retina of the eye and is one of the leading causes of childhood blindness. I remembered Oklyn being tested and the doctor telling us, right after that particular test, that everything was looking just fine. This, however, was not the case with Koraly, as the doctor told the nurse that he would like to retest her eyes in two weeks. Once the nurse told me that there was going to be another visit from the ophthalmologist, I immediately started to question her but she didn't know much more than what she had already told me. Naturally, I started to panic and imagine the worst. I started to think that Koraly would need surgery that could only be done at the Voulder General Children's Hospital, or that she could even be blind. With my hormones bouncing up and down like a yoyo after the recent delivery, I was still very emotionally fragile. I think that Koraly's good health was making the situation less stressful for everyone else, but I still hadn't finished dealing with the disappointment with the first pregnancy. Patience is definitely one of the virtues that parents need when they have a premature baby, but by then I just had none left. I had used all of it with Oklyn while waiting to see if her development would be affected by what they had seen on the second MRI. That is why I could not just sit down, enjoy my baby Koraly while waiting to see what would happen at her next eye appointment. Instead, I was spending my time imagining the worst. The ophthalmologist came back twice, two weeks between each appointment just as he said he would, and at our last visit he finally told us that things had resolved themselves, as they do in most of the cases. I was relieved, but could not understand why in situations like this, the communication between doctors, nurses and parents could not be better. Why were they not explaining what they had found to the parents? Were they too busy? It's no wonder why as parents we were always turning to the Internet to find an explanation of what was going on.

During Koraly's stay in the Everwood Queen's Hospital nursery, I was haunted by a nagging fear that she would need to go back to the Voulder General Children's Hospital for some reason or other. The Voulder General Children's Hospital was great, but going back there would mean that my baby girl was not doing well. On March 29th, my fears became a reality. Koraly needed an inguinal hernia repaired, just like her sister. I could not believe it. Going back to Voulder this time was going to be a little more difficult with Oklyn at home. It meant that one of us would stay home and the other one would accompany Koraly and spend the time she would need for recovery at the Voulder

General Children's Hospital. It made sense that I should go with her as I was breastfeeding and I could provide what she would need during her stay. All this worried me as I really didn't feel strong enough to go through this ordeal alone. What if a complication arose and I was all by myself?

When we got to the Voulder General Children's Hospital the night of March 31st, I was approached immediately by a doctor who wanted Koraly to undergo her second MRI, just as Oklyn did when she went for her hernia repair. I am not exactly sure what made me make this decision, but I refused to have it done. I was worried that perhaps that they'd find out that there was a change in her white brain matter. Moreover, after all our needless worry over the misleading results of Oklyn's MRI, I had no faith in that study. Oklyn was a great example that what they had seen didn't amount to much. I was not ready to let them give me bad news about Koraly's future, especially information that could not totally be explained. I wanted to take Koraly home, and this time really enjoy her and not have to worry every minute about her growing up. Apart from the hernia, she was healthy and developing well so there was no point in having her go through this. I decided, however, that I would return for her eighteen-month and three-year follow-ups, just to show them how well she was doing. A MRI with inconclusive results did not interest me and, to be honest, the thought of dealing with bad news all by myself scared me.

We flew back to Everwood three days later. Once we got to the Everwood Queen's Hospital nursery, we were told that Koraly was ready to come home! In order to receive the official discharge, she had to pass the car seat test and needed to continue to gain weight. I was positive that she would do just fine. Was I ready for her homecoming? To my surprise, I was not yet totally ready. I was still very dependent on the cardiac and respiratory monitor, and I knew that I was this mom who would never be ready to take a baby home after spending three months in an intensive care nursery.

Koraly was discharged from the Everwood Queen's Hospital nursery on April 15th weighing five pounds and eight ounces. She had been hospitalised for a total of seventy-seven days, twenty days less than Oklyn, and she weighed only one ounce less than her sister had at the time of her discharge. Due to her stronger start, Koraly was doing so much better than her sister. She had had a shorter stay in the hospital, had experienced less complications and she barely needed medication.

The morning before Koraly was discharged, a nurse asked me if it made a difference or not, knowing before delivering that I was afflicted with the disease. I pondered her interesting question. I had no doubt that it was good to know in advance that I had the disease as it gave Koraly a stronger start, but it also created an insecurity, and a loss of control and trust of my own body. I also believe that knowing didn't help me overcome my fears and constant worries. I told her, however, that I preferred to be the one suffering rather than my baby girl.

Koraly was a very bad sleeper, just like her sister. I was told that because their stomachs were still premature, it was very hard for them to settle and sleep. However, we did notice that she was a very content baby, smiling and cooing early, and that she was gaining weight just like a full-term baby. She was still keeping us very busy because she was also involved with the Infant Development Program and was being monitored by a nurse. I was worried about her, but not as much as I had been with Oklyn. I think I was able to enjoy Koraly more, and I don't know if it was because I was just too busy to worry or if it was because she seemed very healthy. I was not constantly focusing on her development and on how she would do in the future. We didn't wait very long to take Koraly to restaurants, stores or friends' houses, as she was always exposed to her sister's germs anyway. Oklyn, the big sister, was by this time attending a daycare three days a week. Koraly's needs added to our busy household activities. We were busier because we were dealing with two children under the age of two, but it seemed like it was a very healthy busy. I was finally going to be able to enjoy my maternity leave and maybe even find the peace I had been looking for since this whole adventure started.

The Plus and the Minus

Although I still sometimes wake up thinking that this was all a bad dream, I am quickly brought back to reality when I hear my two beautiful girls chattering away. It was quite a journey and it is still not over. Will it ever be, really? Once a mom, always a mom! This adventure truly changed my life and who I am. Of course the greatest changes were positive: their names are Oklyn and Koraly. However, I have noticed negative changes in myself. Over the past three years I've become very insecure. I have obsessive thoughts that make me feel mentally exhausted because I always see the worst in every happy situation.

On the positive side, I can say that this adventure has made me realise that life is very fragile and that I should enjoy every moment of it. My life went from being healthy and happy to lying down on a hospital bed not knowing if my baby and I would survive. It really taught me to celebrate life and to honour each of my girls' milestones. I make time on a weekly basis to recognize how fortunate Mack and I are to have two beautiful, normal developing girls. I can't stop questioning myself and wondering how we would have gotten through something so difficult if the outcome would have been unfavourable. How would we have coped had our daughters not developing well or were unhealthy? I have learned to be compassionate to people who are not as fortunate as we are. I now look at my students differently, and always try to show empathy towards parents who are having a difficult time raising their children. I am also trying not to be judgemental, as we never know what is lurking in some child's past that makes him or her behave in a certain way.

My mom told me that the last three years happened for a reason. There were, and still are, times when I don't know why this ordeal was sent my way, but it certainly brought some life-changing attitudes that I would not have developed if I had not experienced these two challenging births. My thoughts on marriage, love, friendship, and family got shaken, but only to make me realise what is really important in life. Over the course of this dramatic experience, my family and my friends gave us amazing support, and without them it would have been extremely difficult to cope. These experiences have taught me to take care of those dear to us and to maintain our friendships even in times when I just feel like isolating myself. These wonderful people were there for us, and I understood that they only wanted to help us and to share our pain. Over time, it became easier to give them an update and to cry with them and let them hold us. I can truly say that my family and friends helped us adopt the right attitude in such a painful situation. I am happy that I accepted their phone calls and e-mails and that I included them in our lives, because it allowed them to stand beside us when we needed support to face our difficult decisions.

I would be lying if I said that these experiences didn't affect our marriage. We each deal differently with stress, but I can now say that through this adventure our marriage emerged stronger than ever before. Stress and lack of sleep is a very bad combination when attempting to maintain a healthy marriage. I am no longer the self-confident woman Mack married, and as for Mack, sometimes it was difficult for me to understand his reactions when facing hard times. When handling complex situations, I obsess with negative thoughts. Mack, on the other hand, tries to avoid the problem in the hope that it will disappear. There is no doubt in my mind, however, that the combination of our personalities helped us go through these two births without totally giving up. He was there to remind me that life keeps going on and that obsessing about the outcome was not going to fix our problem. I can now tell young lovers that there is nothing in the world that will prepare them more for marriage than going through a challenging ordeal. Surviving hard times as a couple is what tells you if you are meant to be together or not.

As a result of all this trauma, I have lost my sense of adventure. My daughters' births have made me become this crazy mother who fears everything. For example, when I plan a trip I often have the thought that the plane will crash or that while driving somewhere we will have an accident. When my children are sick, their smallest malaise makes me assume that they are suffering from an incurable disease.

I used to be adventurous, self-confident, fun and patient. I even thought that I was invincible. Now I am more fragile and often find myself lost in my own thoughts. In fact, thinking has become my new hobby, as I can now sit for hours and think about the worst of every situation. People around me tell me that I have become more sensitive. I often get teary-eyed when I speak about my children. I just want to remind the people around me that I have scars now that won't totally heal, and I don't think they will heal at all unless I start dealing with the fears and the worries that these two births brought to my life. I believe that I will have to stop brushing my feelings away and deal with the problem. I have been feeling mentally exhausted over the past few years because of the stress that this journey has brought to my life. Now is a good time to sit up and deal with all these feelings. I know that I will never get pregnant again, never deliver a premature baby again and never again have to call the NICU home. After spending six months of my life in a NICU, I can now tell you what it is to have a miracle baby. Having a miracle baby is delivering a full-term, healthy baby. I can barely look at pregnant women anymore. I can barely congratulate a pregnant mom because I know what could be hiding behind this round belly. Instead of feeling happy for this expectant mother, I am frightened about all the painful things that might be in store for her.

It would be wrong to complete this book without mentioning that the most important thing that kept us going over this difficult and uncertain time was the unconditional love we had for our daughters right from the beginning and the hope that our girls would be just fine. I could not tell you what I thought "fine" meant during this ordeal, but there was this unconditional love that was forcing us and helped us to wake up every morning. We did have moments of huge disappointments and inconsolable tears, but we kept ourselves surrounded with positive people and we continued asking questions until answers were found. We trusted the specialists, but we also had to make our decisions based on what was best for us and what we believed in. Over these years we became not only parents, but also advocates for our daughters, and we tried to base our decisions on what we felt was best for all of us. We learned to put our trust in the future rather than solely on the various doctors' reports. It is sometimes hard to believe that Oklyn's APGAR was zero at birth, one at five minutes, three at ten minutes, and that now she is going through the terrible twos just like any other typical two-year-old.

I call my children sweethearts, mes petits amours, mes petits trésors, mes petits cocos, my little pumpkins. My friends call them my little miracles. The taxpayers call them the million dollar babies. I know for sure that if any taxpayers had been in my shoes, they would consider that every penny spent on these beautiful children was worth it. I will always remember the conversation a doctor and I had as I was waiting for the Infant Transport Team to come and get Koraly for the very last time before coming home. I told her that my million dollar baby was on her way home. She gave me the kindest smile and the most comforting pat on the back and said "It was all worth it." I agreed, and let a tear roll down my cheek.

From where we live in Everwood, we can see the planes

starting their descent to the airport and once in a while I will recognise one with the Infant Transport Team on board. I point to the plane and tell my daughters that there is "un avion" on its way to help someone in need or maybe even save a life just as it did for them. Then I just can't stop smiling and feeling fortunate that we live in Canada, a country where my two daughters got the medical care they needed to in order to survive, to be healthy, and to develop into the sweethearts they are today. Try as I may, I will never be able to adequately thank everyone for the care that we received over these past years. I will never be able to find words strong enough to express what is in my heart. I will only be able to write it in a card here and there that I will drop off at the nursery, to our paediatrician and even to the specialists' offices. Here is a note that I wrote to the specialists in Voulder after they delivered Koraly.

> *We were hoping for thirty-seven weeks, but we only got twenty-eight! However, twenty-eight weeks followed by the best care from our doctors means so much more. It was another very scary experience, but with your help and the help of your team we got through the first step - the delivery. The road will not be smooth for our new baby girl, but we have been here before. We now know the routine and we also know how rewarding the outcome can be. One of you told me, during an appointment, not to end this pregnancy, because the joy that I would get seeing my daughter grow up would be way better than having any regret for the loss of my child. I can al-*

ready see that you were right. Please keep researching, studying and investigating so that one day women like myself can have a stress-free and healthy pregnancy.

Acknowledgments

I would like to thank Roxanne Dauncey for her many hours of hard work spent on editing this story. Her ideas to make this book more compelling were very appreciated and so was the glass of wine we would share after each get-together.

Another thank you goes to Betty Jakel also for her time spent at editing this story and for her generous ideas that she shared with me in regards of making this write-up easier for the reader to understand.

I could not write an acknowledgment without thanking my husband, family and friends who gave me all the support I needed to go through this ordeal. I am grateful for every little attention.

A special thank you goes to my friend Lynn Shanko who kept encouraging me to write this story. Thank you, Lynn, for your kind words whenever I would send you a page or two to read because it helped me realise one of my many dreams, to write a book.

Made in the USA
Monee, IL
04 November 2026

67387511R00056